MW00479746

WIDOW

How Grief Made Room For Happiness

WISDOM

*With "Reader Invitations"
to personalize experiences shared by the author*

RUTH E. RIGBY

All sorrows can be borne if you put them in a story or tell a story about them.

Isac Dinesen

One small year
It's been an eternity
It's taken all of me to get here

Shawn Colvin
from song "One Small Year"

READERS' RESPONSE:

- "This is a go-to book for older widows."

- "I had the same chills reading it a second time."

- "The author writes about things I haven't read before. It blew me away!"

- "I loved the song lyrics. They shifted the mood in a refreshing and fun way."

- "This is a book that comes from the heart of a woman who knows of what she speaks!"

- "The author struggled with her identity as an older widow, and emerged with grace, confidence, and purpose. Let her experience with grief bring you to a point where you can feel those things, too."

- "I'm not a big reader, but this book was so interesting. It read like a novel."

- "I love this book. The insights of the journey to find your self will inspire women to know how to move forward. Just wish I had a book like this to help me when I first became a widow."

- "The pages to write down thoughts are priceless. The kite artwork is great, and I love the poems and music lyrics that soothed my memories."

- "This book gave me peace of mind. It helped me understand being a new widow, and that over time I was going to be OK."

- "The author supports other widows by sharing how she coped and made positive changes after losing her own husband."

AUTHOR'S INVITATION TO READ:

- It's okay to cry. Grief is a room that dwells within us. Sometimes we go there.

- I already knew what grief was. I was living it. I wanted to know how to get out of it!

- I wanted a book with laser focus on "How did you live? What did you do? How long did it take?" I wanted a story around those questions.

- How does grief make room for happiness? <u>Widow Wisdom</u> answers that question.

- This book is for every other older widow who, like me, wants to live beyond grief and seeks to know how.

- Think of your "widow identity" as only the time between the death of your husband and the time you intentionally declare it is time to act.

- What you will work for is the gradual transition from your "widow identity" to a life that is not defined by loss. That is what this book is about.

- I had not accepted my own day by day lifestyle death—a wife to widow life. I knew how to be wife; I did not know how to be widow—alone.

- Initially, what I needed was another widow to "emotionally dwell" with me—a wise woman—a woman who understood deeply because she had lived my experience. I never had that. This book imparts the wisdom I sought.

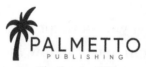

PALMETTO
PUBLISHING

Charleston, SC
www.PalmettoPublishing.com

WIDOW WISDOM
Copyright © 2021 by Ruth E. Rigby

Paperback: 978-1-63837-164-9
Hardcover: 978-1-63837-165-6
eBook: 978-1-63837-166-3

FOR MY AUNT LOENA
a widow at forty-five
I did not know then what I know now.
Through it all, you ended up making us laugh
and showing us a good time.
We still tell your stories.

FOR NEWLY WIDOWED WOMEN
whose husband shockingly died during the
COVID-19 pandemic of 2020
maybe for Jessica, Mary, Denise, Katy, Brenda,
Elizabeth, Martha, Rose, and all the unnamed X
Your loss symbolizes a world's grief.

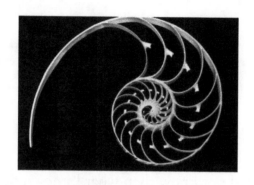

The Chambered Nautilus
(from stanza three)

Still, as the spiral grew
He left the past year's dwelling for the new,
Stole with soft step its shining archway through,
Built up its idle door,
Stretched in his last found home,
And knew the old no more.

by Oliver Wendell Holmes

TABLE OF CONTENTS

CHAPTER 1

SEARCHING FOR WISDOM

The average age to become a widow is fifty-nine, so I consider myself fortunate to have made it longer than that—but not by much. I was sixty-two when I was widowed. Even the word "widow" sounds so gloomy with its whispered "W" and its painful "Oh" ending. It's the right sounding word to parallel the emptiness, loss, and pain an older woman faces after her husband dies. It is a word that embodies hurt.

I know what grief is. I lived it. You know what grief is, too, even though you may not understand it. Either you are living with it clouding endless days and nights, or recovering from it sucking away joy and peace.

What I did not know was how to live my newly widowed life. No other widowed woman shared her shattered life experiences with me. (I only knew two.) Even my own mother could not offer a wisdom I had expected. It was just too personal. This book imparts the wisdom I sought.

Books offered to me by my grief counselor, although sincere, were too devotional and prayerful. They did not delve into the pith of my grief. I sought other books, but I was not ready for a technical analysis of grief, or psychological journaling workbook, or advice to navigate funeral and finances. Some books I browsed were just too long for my short, jittery attention span. Maybe save for later. Many books, heavy on grief, served as self-cathartic healing, which was fine for the writer, but placed little emphasis on the reader's need to step beyond grief. I wanted a book with laser focus on "How did you live? What did you do? How long did it take?" I wanted a story around those questions.

I found only one book of interest, one written by a prestigious writer, so I knew her telling would be precise and crafted. I started with Joan Didion's <u>The Year of Magical Thinking</u>, her mournful memoir about the one year following her husband's deadly heart attack as she routinely served dinner in their Manhattan apartment. "Ordinary". I winnowed out the other tragedy of Didion's one year, the critical hospitalization of her only child, a daughter. It was overwhelming for me to read that part, too, newly widowed, while at the same time, navigating and advocating in a medical world, taking charge of her daughter's fight to live. How heartbreaking! Didion's experience was a lesson in how a woman braved a passage that most women will face, and few men will ever have to experience.

But, I needed Didion's story to continue past her one year, although I knew why she ended. "It's finished." I already knew what grief was. I was living it. I wanted to know how to get out of it! I took the bits of wisdom I could—her stories from the past and her brave onward march through crisis—to understand a newly widowed life, but my unanswered question stuck with me. "How does grief make room for happiness?" Widow Wisdom answers that question.

When my husband died, life as I knew it did not exist, and I knew it never would. I already knew my husband was going to die. No year of magical thinking gave me thought that death could somehow be erased and life rewritten. My past was filled with memories. My present was grief-filled loss. My future was filled with uncertainty.

What I discovered over time, however, was that living beyond grief equated to reinventing my life. LIVING BEYOND GRIEF EQUATED TO REINVENTING MY LIFE. I only realized this by analyzing my own twenty month life-after- death experience. I did not sit down and create flow charts of a hopeful future. I did not invoke mental imagery of a hopeful future. I did not pray for a hopeful future. Rather, my hopeful future evolved over time because my willingness to make changes and live differently made it possible. Like the chambered nautilus, I gradually "left the past year's dwelling for the new". I purposefully created room for happiness.

This book is for every other older widow who, like me, wants to live beyond grief and seeks to know how. One way to know is from another woman's experience. Each chapter of <u>Widow Wisdom:How Grief Made Room for Happiness</u> is my widow story of how to reinvent a life so the new can come in. It takes inner strength, self-reliance, and bravery, but it also takes time. My uncertain future became a retrospective, encouraging you to also make room for happiness.

Think of your "widow identity" as only the time between the death of your husband and the time you intentionally declare it is time to act. <u>Widow Wisdom</u> identifies 7 purposeful actions mindful of your happiness. Whether or not you claim these actions for yourself is up to you, but there is NO DOUBT, at some point you must act! No one else can do it for you. Yes, be hopeful, but also act; it proves your will to live beyond grief.

Because no two experiences are the same, I have included "Reader Invitations" for you to reflect on specific stories from you and your husband's life together—places, people, events—and to also reflect on the actions you are willing to take to reinvent your life. Invitations are a way for you to personalize my experiences into your very own. I have also included literature connections that reveal life's truth and speak universally to the human condition.

"Preach! Write! Act! Do anything save to lie down and die!"

Hester Prynne to Rev. Dimmesdale
<u>The Scarlet Letter</u> by Nathaniel Hawthorne

254

Hope is the thing with feathers
that perches in the soul,
and sings the tune without the words,
and never stops at all,
And sweetest in the gale is heard;
And sore must be the storm
That could abash the little bird
That kept so many warm.
I've heard it in the chillest land,
And on the strangest sea;
Yet, never, in extremity,
It asked a crumb of me.

by Emily Dickinson

CHAPTER 2

REMEMBERING OUR STORIES

Call him Adam.

I knew that I wanted to be happy again. For that to manifest, I resignedly accepted I had to create changes in my life. This sounds like an abandonment of the love and shared life with Adam, my husband, but I assure you it was not. In fact, only in retrospect did I even know I had actually reinvented my life, because the steps were so gradual. It is this process of reinventing a life—inviting the new to come in— that will move you from widow's grief to a happier life.

Our stories did not die.

Before the cancer illness that ended Adam's life, I described myself as living a charmed life. We married at thirty-two and thirty-four. I always called our marriage day the middle—the middle of our lives, the middle of the year, the middle of the month, the middle of the week, and the middle of the day—the middle.

It was a second marriage for both of us, and by choice we had no children. That allowed us to live an adventurous life, carefree and spontaneous all of our nearly thirty year marriage. Adam died at sixty-three. I had just turned sixty-two.

From our first meeting, everything about Adam was unique. The day we met he turned to me and asked, "Would you like to go fly a kite?" So carefree, we shopped at a toy store, bought two kites, drove to Atlanta's Piedmont Park and flew kites. It was a gorgeous and warm February thirteenth. Right after that, on our first official date, we sailed on Lake Lanier, my introduction to what would become our boating life.

After months of dating and even geographical separation, one dusk-lit evening we walked a garden path, sat on a big rock, and talked. Adam asked what I planned to do for Thanksgiving. I told him that I would be visiting my family in Florida. "Well, I guess I should go with you so your parents can meet their new son-in-law." I was joyously stunned. That was his marriage proposal to me.

When planning our honeymoon, Adam asked, "Would you rather have a one week honeymoon or a six week honeymoon?" You can already predict my answer. His mother gifted us a new pop-up Scamper camper, and on the afternoon of our simple garden wedding, we took off for Savannah then camped our way down the east coast of Florida all the way to Key West, returning up the west coast of Florida to Atlanta.

We knew we wanted to live in Southwest Florida, prime sailing waters protected by barrier islands. So we packed up and moved there. Boating was a big part of our lives all our years together. We spent countless days on secluded island beaches, as well as many overnights anchored to a moonbeam, listening to sounds of dolphin exhaling and fish jumping.

If an illness preceded death, it is likely that stories were shared as part of the ritual of dying. From a hospice bed, Adam told his own story of how his high school letter jacket, as a result of cleaning out, had been given away while he was at college. He told how he felt such disappointment, because he had lettered in swimming and had been awarded a pin for winning state.

All those years ago, but he still remembered his prized possession. All six of us sitting near his bed remarked we had no idea. We had never heard that story. My brother, Charles, acted immediately to contact the athletic director at Adam's former high school in Ohio. Staff over-nighted Adam a Findley High School letter with a swimming award pin attached, and included a heartfelt note and best wishes. I love my brother for doing that.

The stories go both ways. Rick and Debbie recalled family stories of growing up as kids. Adam was their big brother. Trish, the baby sister, told stories with more adult experiences. They bonded even more closely during the dying months because of her care visits, empathetic nature, and their frank talks.

Some stories were more private, like when Rebekah would call to talk and pray with Adam, or when Rosemary would call with a funny story to cheer him up, or when Charles or Tony or Rick called to engage in some man talk.

Adam could have told his story of buying a Bristol 32 sailboat in Mystic, Connecticut, then motoring his way down the intercoastal waterway to Ft. Lauderdale before taking off for the Bahamas—the Abacos—for a year of cruising.

Or he could have told the story about his love of flying, how he learned at a young age, and how as an older man bought his own vintage J-3 Cub, and how it won an award in its class at the Sun 'N Fun airshow. How he would fly low over the meandering Peace River, or fly over the Gulf of Mexico coastline. How one day he flew inland over farmland and spotted a grass landing strip near a house and barn, so he landed. How he met the owner and they struck up a friendship. It is not every day that a stranger lands an airplane in your backyard!

I think one of the most remarkable stories of Adam's life is his first-hand account of witnessing the Kent State shootings while he was a college student there. Because I think his story is such an important part of American history, I have included it at the end of this book. Postpone that reading, because your laser focus right now is on understanding how to live a newly widowed life that is not defined by grief.

You have stories, too. The day you married was filled with hopes and dreams; filled with romance, emotion, and passion. Most likely you started a family and nurtured them through the early years to graduations and their own mature adult lives. The loss of your husband now stops you in your tracks and the uncertainty of the future looms. The grief is inconsolable at times and the feeling of emptiness pervades.

The stories you tell reveal the life your husband lived, the life you shared as husband and wife, and his life as son, brother, father, and friend. Death brings back memory stories to comfort you. Embrace them. Hold them close to your heart. It's an important step in the process to release your grief, and a baby step to reinvent your life. Your memory stories did not die.

The past is never dead. It is not even past.
William Faulkner

READER INVITATION: Think about marrying your husband. How did you meet? What attracted you to him? What special place did you honeymoon? Think about your life together. What did you enjoy doing together? What made you laugh? What is a favorite memory story you tell? What is a special story others tell? What are stories your husband told? What one story do you think will live on?

NOW WRITE YOUR STORY:

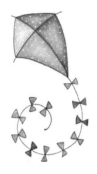

The weeks wrapped around death are when your family and friends will come to you, even if they do not know what to do. Let them, even if *you* do not know what to do. It is part of the story.

Rosemary, my sister, drove six hundred twenty miles to stay with me through the final hours, and kept my head above water those first days after. We sat with our feet in a bubbling basin of water distracted by a pedicure while I babbled random ideas about a memorial service. All the time she was writing notes and keeping the tone lighthearted, as only she could do. Alone, I would have been at home stuck and toiling over the plans. I love her very much.

By the day she left, I knew what I had to do— arrange a gallery exhibit of Adam's life at Leoma Lovegrove's Gallery and Gardens, a funky place where Adam and I purchased art and browsed to the sound of Beatles music. Provide gathering food and drink, create a garden artwalk of canvas photos and video, end with eulogy, poem, song, prayer, Isaiah 40:31 scripture, and a comfort message. That was the plan.

Like changing shifts at the widow house, my other sister, Rebekah, arrived at the airport the same day Rosemary left. Her diligence in making sure my house was in order, while at the same time occupying my time with thoughtful encouragement and strong faith, lifted my spirits. Her practical approach to details marched me through the end of the week to the day I brought home the urn of cremains. I love her very much.

Friends will also be there for you. They will mail a card, call, text, bring food, run errands, clean your house, walk your dogs, deliver a mocha frappe, pour you a glass of wine, and just be with you. My friends are dear to me. Even two cousins traveled to spend only one hour with me.

Family and friends grieve, too. Yet somehow their strength is greater than yours, because they have been able to reach out to you despite feeling their own loss. Who comforts them?

The last two pieces, the memorial service and burial, put a period on the death event. Not a question. Not an exclamation. A final period. It is after the death events that your life starts with a question mark. You were wife. Now you are widow. How do I live my newly widowed life? Your goal is to leave your "widow identity" behind by taking actions that help you reinvent your life as an exclamation of happiness!

I counted ninety artfully written names in Adam's memorial guest book. At the end of the evening, each person received a free ice cream from Great Licks which was next door to the gallery. I think ice cream was a little bit of comfort for them to end the evening. Don't you?

What is a funeral except to comfort the living, to eulogize a life—to speak of accomplishments, relationships, love—to tell life stories? Even after the funeral, memory stories are told.

Nurture your story experiences. Tell them or hold them in your heart because they ease the grief and loss. Again, it's an important step in the process to release your grief, and a baby step to reinvent your life.

Great Licks – Queenie's Ice Cream

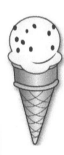

Receive a FREE gourmet ice cream treat from Great Licks, next door to Lovegrove Gallery.

Adam enjoyed stopping at Great Licks and it is his treat to you as you leave this evening.

Thank you for being here.

CHAPTER 3

ACCEPTING TWO DEATHS

Part of growing out of grief is the acceptance that life as it was no longer exists. My husband died. He is gone. He is not coming back. That's a harsh realization, and even more shocking is that it happens with his last breath. Breath in. Breath out. Gone.

The only other time I experienced this same finality was the day I walked into our home for the first time by myself after Adam died. Family from out of town had stayed during the dying. Napa, California; Atlanta, Georgia; Pensacola, Florida; Stow, Ohio. No mother. No father. Only brothers and sisters gathered for our sacred and profound event—a passage. So my experiencing being alone in our house for the very first time was eight days after Adam died.

With Adam's two dogs in the car with me, I drove my sister, Rebekah, to the airport. I wished that she could have stayed longer. That same afternoon I would bring Adam's cremains home. I wanted the dogs with me because I would drive from the airport directly to the funeral home. Adam had often re-marked how Google kept him company and would lie next to him on his bed on bad days. Merlin's energy, antics, and happy dance made him laugh. I felt strongly that Adam's dogs should have their own part in the ritual of dying. This would be it.

I left the car running with the air conditioner on for the dogs. I walked inside, sat at a conference table, listened to the solemn voice of the funeral director, completed some paperwork, signed a document, and left carrying a burled wood urn. I sat with it in my lap and quietly cried while I drove six miles home. I cradled it with my left arm. I could not let go. Nothing could have prepared me for this substitution.

The dogs knew something, because there was no barking and no happy dance. They were quiet and still. Google, who always sat in the front seat beside me, lay down in the back seat, his head near the console, looking up at me. Merlin sat in the front seat, alternately looking at me and out the front window, always the co-pilot.

The dogs followed me into the house. I talked to them about how they gave comfort and joy to Adam, but I never spoke his name, because they knew and recognized his name. I did not want them to anticipate seeing Adam. I told them what I was doing while I placed the urn on a narrow table under our favorite blue artwork—a vast ethereal modern sky painted with prominent clouds and a stairway of cubed shapes stepped into a pool of sparkling water. We bought it at a gallery on Canyon Road in Santa Fe. If ever there was a heaven, this painting could be it. I placed my hands on each of the dogs' heads; we blessed his urn. This space became a sacred altar for the next weeks.

The feeling of emptiness in the house was overwhelming. I knew Adam was gone, but now, for the first time, even his energy was gone. Final. It was as if the house had been sucked dry. It was a vacuum with his wife and two dogs wandering room to room seeking some sign.

There is no transition from married life to widowed life. It is immediate. That is one reason it is so very difficult to accept. You walk through that door and you are instantly alone. There is no conversation, no dinner companion, no hug and kiss. For my mother it was no one to hold her hand. I do not need to list these losses, because you are already experiencing them. You know this part so well because you are newly trying to live through it. What you will work for is the gradual transition from your "widow identity" to a life that is not defined by loss. That is what this book is about.

You may be unaware that in addition to grieving your husband's death, you are also grieving the loss of your own life that no longer exists. Accepting dual loss is a necessary step to live beyond grief. Grief will gradually weave into the fabric of your life, but will sometimes become that noticeable loose thread—a Lazarus snagged by some marker association.

There are just some things that you will not anticipate being a loss. Of course, all the day to day marriage interactions are gone. That is a foregone loss. But there will be a significant lifestyle loss, too. For me, it was the loss of our boating life. We had always owned a boat. We were on the water and anchored at an island beach nearly every week of the year. We lived in southwest Florida where winters are warm. Only infrequent cold or a rainy day prevented us from boating. I had to accept my boating life ended.

My husband died. He is gone. He is not coming back. Actually, that he is not coming back may be only part truth. A few weeks after he died, I saw my husband. I was asleep, but awoke to a distinct presence. I immediately sat up and saw Adam standing a few feet from my bed, smiling at me. I exclaimed his name, "Adam!" It was that real! But as quickly as I voiced his name the sight of him vanished. I tried to will him back to me. I questioned afterwards, if I had been silent, would he have lingered? His smile was so beautiful. I saw him in full health, muscular, handsome and tall. I will never forget it.

A friend from my past told me she experienced a similar event, waking and seeing her deceased husband. I share this deeply personal experience with you because if it has not already happened to you, it probably will. It did not alarm me. Instead, it affirmed for me that there is a form of life after death that manifests to console grief. I cannot interpret how you will react to this phenomenon, but without a doubt it will be a positive experience.

All the longing to see Adam one more time did happen for me. Even for a brief moment, I was comforted and felt that Adam's presence would always be with me. Although I once had a vivid dream about him, I have never seen him since that one appearance, but it was significant enough that I know his spirit is still part of my life.

That was affirmed to me once again six years later—not by the sight of him, but from the sound of his voice speaking to me. Standing in the beamed loft of a log home, with light filtering through trees and a view of mountains, I clearly heard Adam's voice speak to me, "If you want this house, you can have it. I gave it to you." It was not a thought; it was his voice.

It is the sound of Adam's voice that continues to be a loss for me. For the longest time I would call his cell phone just to hear him speak. I regret not recording his voice because over time, its clarity has diminished. I remember less and less the sound of his voice. That I heard him speak to me six years later diminished this loss.

You might feel unsettled as you read this section. It *is* incredulous, but for me, seeing and hearing have been two very real sensory perceptions of Adam's presence since he died.

Acceptance that your life will never be the same after the death of your husband is a necessary step forward in your journey toward reinventing a life. The time it takes depends on your strength and, I think, whether death came at the end of a long illness, or death came in a sudden tragic manner. Only you will know this.

In some circumstances, perhaps even the imminent signs of your husband's impending death could not be accepted. *If I do not accept his medical problem, then he will not die any time soon.* Following is a literary example to understand this type of pre-death non-acceptance:

In the early 20th century story "A Journey" by Edith Wharton, a wife travels by train with her dying husband. Following "six weeks of mild air" in Colorado, his doctors consent to their journey home to New York. Wharton describes this wife's non-acceptance of her husband's impending death—how she "dressed the truth" and slipped into making "next year's plans".

"There were moments, indeed, when warm gushes of pity swept away her instinctive resentment of his condition, when she still found his old self in his eyes as they groped for each other through the dense medium of his weakness. But these moments had grown rare.

Sometimes he frightened her: his sunken expressionless face seemed that of a stranger; his voice was weak and hoarse; his thin-lipped smile a mere muscular contraction. Her hand avoided his damp soft skin, which had lost the familiar roughness of health: she caught herself furtively watching him as she might have watched a strange animal. It frightened her to feel that this was the same man she loved; there were hours when to tell him what she suffered seemed the one escape from her fears. But in general she judged herself more leniently, reflecting that she had perhaps been too long alone with him, and that she would feel differently when they were at home again, surrounded by her robust and buoyant family.

How she had rejoiced when the doctors at last gave their consent to his going home! She knew, of course, what the decision meant; they both knew. It meant that he was to die; but they dressed the truth in hopeful euphemisms, and at times, in the joy of preparation, she really forgot the purpose of their journey, and slipped into an eager allusion to next year's plans."

In spite of the vivid physical images of death's grip on her husband's body, the wife cannot face the truth; she erases it with her "joy of preparation". The story further demonstrates her inability to accept the reality of his impending death.

In contrast to the wife's dismissal and non-acceptance in Wharton's story, is the methodical reality of acceptance by the woman in the following Emily Dickinson poem. Because the poet metaphorically speaks of a domestic chore, "sweeping", I identify the individual as a woman—a woman who speaks of loss not only for herself, but perhaps for her children, too, as indicated by "we". It is a stark image of a woman's response to a death, and her unequivocal acceptance of its finality—her acceptance that life will never be the same.

1108

The bustle in a House
The morning after Death
Is solemnest of industries
Enacted upon Earth—
The Sweeping up the Heart
And putting Love away
We shall not want to use again
Until Eternity--

by Emily Dickinson

Your acceptance of the death of your husband falls somewhere between these two illustrative extremes—dismissal and non-acceptance of death, or an unequivocal acceptance of its finality. I was somewhere in the middle, because even though I had accepted my husband's imminent death, I had not accepted my own day by day lifestyle death—a wife to widow life. I knew how to be wife; I did not know how to be widow—alone.

READER INVITATION: Think about the realization you had the moment your husband died. Did you think about it as the end-not only for your husband, but for you, too? What if you could experience your husband' s presence again? Do you think you have seen or heard your husband speak to you? Have you experienced the presence of your husband in other ways? Over time, and after your grief has settled, are you willing to accept that your life as it was no longer exists? Acceptance that your life will never be the same? List your thoughts about these ideas-your words and phrases- in the form of a poem.

Where do you fall on a scale of acceptance?

I do not accept   full acceptance 5

1	2	3	4	5

NOW WRITE YOUR LIST POEM:

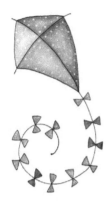

You must accept that your husband died and he is not coming back, and paired with that, you must also accept that the life you had no longer exists. The two are linked. Your grief is for this dual loss. That is why the pain can be almost unbearable at times. Gradually, your grief will become less an assault on your life, and more an acceptance in your life.

Accepting the reality of losing your husband is the hardest step you will take on your journey to reinventing your life. It is also the most important step; otherwise, you will remain a grieving widow with an inability to move forward. You do not want to remain a grieving widow. You want to somehow end up happier.

Psalm 23:4
Yea though I walk through the valley of the shadow of death, I will fear no evil, for Thou art with me…
The Bible

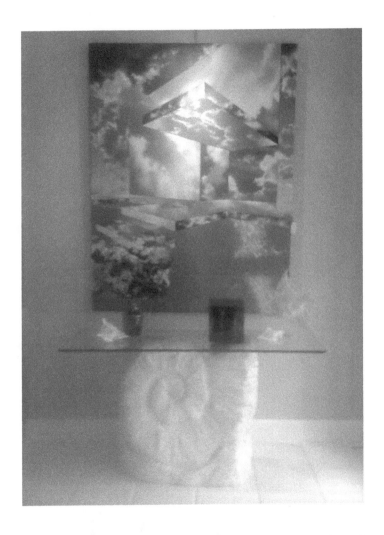

My Altar: "a vast ethereal modern sky painted with prominent clouds and a stairway of cubed shapes stepped into a pool of sparkling water"

CHAPTER 4

RETHINKING GROUP THERAPY

Inevitably because of your loss, you will be informed about grief therapy, either one on one with a counselor, or as part of a group therapy session. A few weeks after Adam died, I went to a group grief therapy session sponsored by the local hospital. I only went because I thought it would help me. It did not help me. I do not recommend a group therapy session as a way to move beyond grief.

The group therapy session was held monthly on the campus of a local hospital. The hospital setting already alerted me to a level of discomfort. I had lost count the number of times I had been to the E.R., sat through an admissions process, and made daily visits to a hospital room, only to endlessly repeat the cycle. The E.R. was so familiar that I knew one E.R. doctor by name. His parting words to Adam after each procedure were, "Keep the faith."

I never wanted to be in a hospital again. I got over it and went anyway, because I was grasping for help. After all, grief therapy was supposed to help. Right?

At least twenty people sat around tables pushed together to form a large rectangle in the meeting room of the hospital. The chair backs were straight up and down as if everyone was at attention. The lighting was bright and harsh, spotlighting each grieving person. The room was whisper quiet—only the sound of murmurs as if not to disturb the dead.

After an initial greeting by the therapist, she welcomed those who were new to the group, so I now knew the majority had attended more than once. This was an ongoing gathering of grievers.

After the welcome, each individual—men and women—were invited by the same therapist to:

Say your name.

Say the name of your deceased loved one.

Tell us the date of your loss.

Tell us why you are here.

Again, I was alerted to a level of discomfort, but I determined to finish what I started. With each individual confession (that's what I called it) there were tears and sometimes quiet sobs. This was not working for me. I was sitting in the middle of grief—of sadness—of hurt. I had put myself in the midst of an entire room full of mourners. I felt trapped; I brace stayed.

When it was my turn to speak the statements, I broke down. I knew I would. I was no different from anyone else in the room. The pain of my loss spilled out tears of sadness even in a room of strangers. What I learned from listening more though, was that some people in this group were there long term—over a year since their loss and they still attended. That alarmed me. Was grief so permanent? And were people so stuck that they could not put grief behind them?

I do not recommend a group therapy grief session to heal your grief. It is not a step forward. Why would you want to hear every other person's sadness and sorrow? You already have enough sadness of your own. Don't invite any more.

It's not that you cannot benefit from others' experiences, but what you want is their experience of moving beyond grief, not their experience of dwelling on grief, of returning to group therapy month after month for a year or more.

In a fragile state, which you are in at the beginning, you need the quiet space of home or the safe comfort of a friend as a gentler means for your emotions to spill. Reading about others' experiences with grief (like you are reading now) will be kinder to your fragile self than seeing drawn faces and hearing trembling voices in a room full of mourners.

I learned from the very beginning that I did not want the burden of other people's grief. I had my own grief to live with. Being in the group setting completely overwhelmed me and added anxiety to my already broken state. Would I be the grieving person sitting in group therapy a year from now saying my name, my husband's name, and why I am here?

I never returned to the group therapy session. What I wanted was to get rid of my grief—to move beyond it. Until then, I would only invite "lovely things" into my life.

Sanctum

I built a tiny garden
In a corner of my heart.
I kept it just for lovely things
And bade all else depart.
And ever was there music
And flowers blossomed fair;
And never was it perfect
Until you entered there.

By Beulah B. Malkin

READER INVITATION: Think about grief support. Were you invited to attend a group therapy session? Did you go? Did you benefit? Or like me, did you feel overwhelmed by grief and anxious that you would remain stuck in grief? Have you gained understanding and the ability to move forward with help from a personal therapist? Are you reading books that help you understand what you are going through? Over time, and after your grief has settled, are you willing to accept that your life as it was no longer exists? Acceptance that your life will never be the same? Sketch or draw how you feel about these ideas.

NOW SKETCH OR DRAW HOW YOU FEEL:

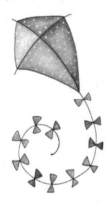

I knew enough about myself after the group therapy experience that I did not want to share my grief with a room full of strangers. What I desired was another widow to "emotionally dwell" with me—a woman wise beyond empathy—a woman who understood deeply because she had lived my experience. I never had that. So my question was the same as when I started my search for understanding how to live my newly widowed life, "How does grief make room for happiness?" I was still searching.

Our hospital at its best: Six days before Adam died, we were in the hospital E.R. for the last time. The familiar doctor, Dr. Schultz, was not attending, but I saw him walk by the open curtain. I hurried to him and asked if he would please, one more time, go to Adam and tell him to "Keep the faith." He did. And Adam did.

It has been seven years. A benefit of time is that looking back I can analyze the steps that helped me move beyond grief to reinvent my life and invite happiness. Being part of a group therapy grief session in a hospital was not one of them.

"It's okay to cry. Grief is a room that dwells within us. Sometimes we go there."

the author, Ruth Rigby

CHAPTER 5

NOT LIVING; DECIDING TO ACT

This is the longest chapter. It is long because these two ideas cannot be separated. They fiercely battle each other, and one of them will win.

For months after Adam died, I would go to work, come home, sit on the lanai, read the news, and play with my two dogs. I did not watch TV or listen to music. I would make myself eat a small meal then go to bed. The winter months made it easy to go to bed early. I just existed. Only Christmas with family interrupted it.

The dogs were Adam's, both unlikely additions to our lives, since the word "dog" had never been uttered by either one of us. Their arrival was a complete surprise to me—a surprise that had to grow on me. Little did I know then, that Google and Merlin would be my best companions, and for a long time, my only source of joy after Adam died. And a part of me thinks Adam knew the dogs would be his enduring gift to me.

I remember eating a lot of cereal and milk and grilled cheese sandwiches. Sometimes dinner was a glass of wine. I remember once stopping by Wendy's to buy chili and a chocolate Frosty. I even posted a picture of my little Wendy's chili dinner on FB, as if that was an event in my life worth sharing. I think about it now, and it makes me sad. It was just plain pitiful that it *was* the only thing in my life worth sharing.

Not living.

That's what I called the eight months after Adam died. I had no motivation to do anything except make myself go to work and manage problems when forced to.

I was a teacher. I remember my first day returning to work after being gone eleven days. Other teachers would see me, smile, and greet me. Their condolences were brief, and I was grateful for that, because hearing words about my loss made me tear up. My emotions were raw. However, it was better that they said something than to ignore my loss.

These teachers had supported me through a long period of certain death. They gave generously to help me when family arrived for Adam's memorial, and several of them attended. Their many, many cards with personal notes had given me comfort. They cared about me. My best friend was one of these teachers.

Adam and I had always celebrated February thirteenth, the day we met and flew kites, so you can imagine the memories that filled my head that day at work—just a few months after he died. This is what I had written in my "progress journal": *February 13. Today I am fragile. I miss Adam the most today.*

The most unlikely caring happened on Valentine's day. After work, a young male teacher arrived at my desk with a chocolate heart and a simple note. I only knew him in passing. He told me he thought this was probably a difficult day for me, and he wanted to cheer me up. I looked at his tattooed arms, his mohawked hair, and his brawny build—an ironic presence for such a tender, caring gift. I had other angels in my life, too, those unexpected, sometimes unknown individuals who appeared once out of nowhere to lift me. Later, you will read about two of them.

This is how my grief manifested during those first months—yes months. I felt like I was in a daze. Hollow. Floating. I felt disconnected from life. Fragile. It was disconcerting to see people living their normal lives—laughing, talking, going places—and me so distanced, as if I observed life from a space above my head, as if I was not even part of my own body. Living a normal life seemed just beyond my reach. I could see it, but I could not participate.

C. S. Lewis, as a widower, described it this way: *"There is a sort of invisible blanket between the world and me. I find it hard to take in what anyone says. Or perhaps, hard to want to take it in."* And you, too, think your own metaphors for how grief makes you feel.

I did what I had to do, sometimes one hour at a time. I had lived like that through Adam's illness, too. By compartmentalizing my life into a day, an hour, or fifteen minute segments, I could accomplish what I had to do and not feel so overwhelmed. You will benefit by knowing this.

I will be brutally honest. Even though you are in the throes of grief with an inability to act for yourself, you have no choice except to also maintain the business of everyday life. Mine was complicated because in addition to working, I managed our commercial properties. This was not new to me, since over a year prior, I had already taken over all of Adam's responsibilities, but managing all this while coping in a grief-fog seemed insurmountable.

A new tenant moved in the same month Adam died, but this particular move-in required me to accomplish tasks that were unfamiliar to me. I solicited help from Mr. Bowen, a contractor friend Adam knew, because I had no knowledge of a schematic for firewall construction, installation of safety lights, and fire safety inspection protocols to meet city code. These were serious tasks and I had to steel myself to manage their completion efficiently and precisely. I also had one tenant move out, and another tenant move in the third month after Adam died. Adam's realtor friend, Mr. Deems, helped with those.

I had no choice but to do these things. Compartmentalizing my tasks helped me bit by bit. It reminded me of the old adage: How do you eat an elephant? One bite at a time. Importantly, I learned to trust individuals who would circle the wagons for me. It was only because Adam had developed loyal and strong business relationships that I knew who to call, and even more, that they wanted to help me.

Also, house repairs that had been on hold for two years could not wait any longer. This was not elected remodeling or redecorating. This was required, under the gun, get it done and done. I had to be WW—Wonder Woman—or, in my case, Wonder Widow with all her superpowers.

After your husband dies, you must rely on your intelligence and prior experience to complete the tasks that seem insurmountable. And these tasks will *all* seem insurmountable if this is the first time you have had to take on these responsibilities by yourself. But you can do it! And you will end up feeling proud of yourself for accomplishing these things, and over time, it gets easier because your confidence grows.

My brother visited over a long weekend to help me understand what needed to be done and to get estimates. Restoration experts, roofer, painter, lawn maintenance crew--all of their work inside and outside my house started the third and fifth month after Adam died.

These are some of the house projects I had to manage, while I simultaneously floated and lived in a grief-fog, and worked full time.

- Gut 15 ft. great room/dining room ceiling, tear out 1,200 sq. ft. tongue and groove boards, replace with drywall, paint

- Select new paint colors, paint walls of great room/dining room (the only fun part)

- Remove and replace two dining room skylights, seal, drywall, paint

- Remove two small sections of metal roof panels, replace

- Remove two small sections of soffit wood, replace, paint

- Tear out chimney base wood trim, replace, redesign flashing around chimney, paint

- Power wash, stain decks

- Remove trees, grind stumps

The most critical repair was the ceiling. Tradesmen were at my house every work day for three weeks to rip out the tongue and groove ash ceiling and complete the restoration project while I was at work. I would meet Jeremy, the project manager, every afternoon to assess the progress, determine any unforeseen problems, and understand the next step. For the most part, it went smoothly. I had hired a reputable restoration company, one Adam had been associated with, so it was more than just another job to them.

I lived in my "bedroom house" with two dogs and visited the kitchen while the main part of the house was in chaos those weeks. Scaffolding, ladders, plastic sheeting barriers, paper walkway runners, tools, and paint cans. Clean up. Project done.

Sometimes you have to figure out how to solve a unique problem all by yourself. It is a problem too peculiar for anyone else. The week before all the house repair jobs started, I had noticed more than once a large horned owl sitting at the top of a tall pine tree when I walked my two dogs in the afternoon. One dog was small.

I had heard owl hoots at night, too. I researched.

- A tuft of feathers creates the horned look

- Has a four and a half foot wing span

- Watches from a high perch

- Swoops down for its prey

- A predator raptor

- Known to sometimes attack small dogs

A dog room off my carport opened to a long, narrow chain link fenced grass area. While I was at work, the dogs were in their room with access to this outside fenced space. I worried that while I was at work the horned owl would attack my small dog when he went outside!

So I drove to Lowe's after work and looked for something to cover the fenced space. I had no idea where to even begin, but I started in the garden section. Who knew there is something called deer net? I also bought four boards long enough to space across the top of the fence, drove home, and constructed a net cover for the outside fenced space. I worked until after dark.

These stories are examples of how I managed the business of day to day life as well as solve unusual problems. You will have to manage problems, too. Some tasks are bigger than others, and you will need to seek help. Some problems are uniquely your own. There are so many more, but in my case these surfaced as the biggest and most unique. Even though grief overpowers your life the first months, you must show grit and determination to solve immediate problems. You do not have a choice in these matters. But one perplexing problem I had, that most people would not, was how to sell a RANS S-7 kit airplane that was sitting in our barn.

Building the airplane was Adam's hobby until he decided to buy a vintage J-3 Cub instead. The frame was constructed, the wings attached. It looked like a big red modern sculpture deserving of a spacious park setting. My selling problem was solved by what I believe to be providential guidance. Remember my angel allusion? Those unexpected, sometimes unknown individuals who appeared once out of nowhere to lift me? Here is a miraculous story:

I had flown to Ohio for my nephew's graduation party five months before my husband died. For some reason my seat was upgraded to business class at check-in. I did not even realize it until I was on the plane looking for my booked seat and the flight attendant told me my seat assignment was up front. So bewildered, I worked my way back—from coach to the first seat of the plane.

I sat by a gentleman who stood to let me sit next to the window. I explained my seat upgrade surprise and having to make my way back to business class. It broke the ice. I had just met Nick. I observed he was reading an aviation magazine, so I started a conversation about flying and the kit plane Adam had been building, but would never finish. Nick had recently completed training for his pilot's license, and was looking to buy a kit plane! He was so interested in my offer to let him see the RANS, that we exchanged contact information. How could this be happening? I was supposed to be sitting in an aisle seat behind the wing, not selling Adam's airplane to a man seated in 1B whom I had just met!

And even more, my artist friend, art gallery owner, Leoma, was on the same plane! We greeted after de-planing at Atlanta airport. In five months I would ask to use her gallery garden for a memorial service, and her minister husband would offer prayers and speak comfort from scripture. "But they that wait upon the Lord shall renew their strength; they shall mount up with wings as eagles; they shall run, and not be weary; and they shall walk, and not faint."

Nick did call me a couple of weeks later to come see the airplane. Adam met Nick for only a brief time in our barn to show the airplane and point out how the parts were labeled and organized in tray compartments. He gave Nick a file box with the paperwork and instruction manuals. It took all the energy Adam had to walk from the house to the barn and converse for twenty minutes.

After a couple of visits and seeing all the plans, files, and perfectly organized mechanical parts—even a new, crated Rotax engine—Nick called to tell me he really preferred to buy a plane with a different seat configuration—side by side, not tandem. But he said, "Please call me later when things settle, and I will help you sell it." I knew what he meant. I did not forget, and made that call to him six months later.

I called Nick January 4. He priced the plane, advertised it in aviation forums and kit magazines, took the calls and e-mails, and answered all the questions. January16 he had an interested buyer who would fly from Salt Spring Island, British Columbia Canada to see the RANS S-7 in the barn at my home in southwest Florida on January 27. He lived 3,375 miles away!!!! Rob loved the airplane, especially because it was an older model, so the next day, January 28, he and Nick worked seven hours to box all the parts, remove the wings, and pack everything ready for shipment. These events all transpired during my third widow month, the same month the major house projects started.

Weeks later, March 18, a large semi-truck arrived at my house and movers loaded Adam's airplane for the long journey to a beautiful place in the world we had read about. It would go through customs in Canada, truck through British Columbia, be loaded onto a ferry to Rob's island, then trailered to his farmhouse property which had its own grass landing strip. If only I could have told this incredibly adventurous part of the story to Adam!

Before the movers arrived, I had placed an envelope into the pouch in front of the pilot's seat. It contained a gold half-heart, my love note, and a picture of Adam posed in front of his J-3 Cub with Patty Wagstaff (the famous aviation aerobatic champion). My exact thoughts were that Adam's spirit would one day fly over the majestic San Juan Islands in his RANS S-7. That would happen because Nick had been my angel.

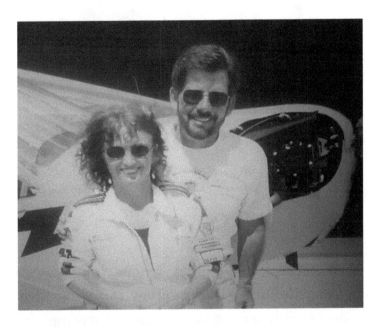

Adam with Patty Wagstaff, the photo I placed in the RANS S-7 before it journeyed to BC Canada

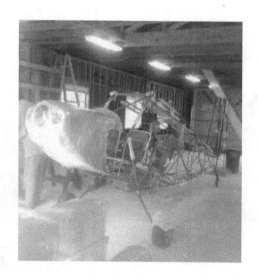

RANS S-7 preparation

I had accomplished multiple serious, complicated, and incredulous tasks during my third and fifth widow month, but even with a sense of accomplishment for putting these arduous tasks behind me, the feeling of loss still invaded my life, especially after the busy-ness of all the projects came to a halt. I figured out why. My "not living" self fiercely battled my undiscovered "deciding to act" self.

The predominant feeling I experienced during months six, seven and eight was that of exclusion. I did not go out much, but when I did, I saw people enjoying themselves. Couples talking. Families going places. Shoppers filling grocery carts. Even the greeter at my Wal-Mart had a purpose.

Life with all its energy, talk, and activity surrounded me. But I stood alone, sat alone, walked alone. Even if I was with a friend, I still felt undercurrents of being alone. I felt isolated, and I also felt a bit unstable, a bit crazy. I felt a more legitimate mental health being alone at home, than feeling alone when surrounded by other people. I felt hollow, unable to insert myself into a normal situation.

I know I was not easy to be with during my "not living" months, because I had nothing positive to contribute. These were the months weighted by my "widow identity". Friendship was one-sided. It didn't matter to my closest friends. They listened. They encouraged. They called. They mailed cards. They gave gifts. They laughed. They asked me to meet for lunch or dinner.

There was the gentle note writer, Donna, and her unexpected drop-by visit with special gifts—one for me and one for the dogs; Carol, the upbeat, enthusiastic encourager, eager to tell the details of golf and travel and island friends and interesting book titles; and the other Carol, easy going hostess and baker, always sharing her homemade chocolate chip cookies and sailing stories.

Cathy, my friend like family, would suggest a brief out of town trip and do all the planning. All I had to do was pack, pay, go. This friend had also said more than once, "Two brains are better than one," when I was dealt a bad hand, and together we fixed it—or at least mended it. She also took care of my dogs when I needed extra help, plus so much more.

Several months later, when grief was slowly releasing its grip on my life, I reaffirmed these closest friendships and became proactive myself to meet regularly for lunch or dinner. I'm a much better friend now. I care about their lives and would do anything to help them. These are the friends who stuck with me when my life was crashing— friends who never gave up on me, and knew that I would one day be in a happy place.

Probably the most vivid and accurate description of how I felt during my battle between "not living" and "deciding to act" comes from the short story "The Open Boat" by Stephen Crane. It is based on a true life experience January 2, 1897 when Crane, a correspondent, on his way by steamer to Cuba, is forced to abandon the sinking "Commodore" after it hits a sandbar. He and three other crew crowd into a small dinghy and struggle for thirty hours toward shore near Ponce Inlet at Daytona Beach, Florida. One of them would drown in the surf. "Not living."

The correspondent finds himself fighting for his life, drifting aimlessly, being violently tossed, bailing water, contemplating death. When he realizes he is in sight of the shore, his hopes improve. He sees people on the beach walking, running near the shore. One man is continuously waving something.

The correspondent thinks these people will certainly help rescue him. Instead, they are tourists going about the happiness of their beach day oblivious to his desperation. He is at the point of drowning, yet so near the shore he can even see that the man on the shore is waving his black coat. The correspondent's dialogue with his fellow boat mates vividly portrays his desperation:

"Funny they don't see us."

"Look! There's a man on the shore!"

"Where?"

"There! See 'im?" See 'im?"

"Yes, sure! He's walking along."

"Now he's stopped. Look! He's facing us!"

"He's waving at us!"…

"There comes something up the beach."

"What the devil is that thing?"

"Why it looks like a boat."

"No, it's on wheels."

"Well that must be the life-boat. They drag them along shore on a wagon."

"That's the life-boat, sure."

"No, by ------, it's—it's an omnibus."

"I tell you it's a life-boat."

"It is not! It's an omnibus. I can see it plain. See? One of those big hotel omnibuses."

"By thunder, you're right. It's an omnibus, sure as fate. What do you suppose they are doing with an omnibus? Maybe they are going around collecting the life-crew, hey?"...

"Oh, say there isn't any life-saving station there. That's just a winter resort hotel omnibus that has brought over some of the boarders to see us drown."

"If I am going to be drowned—if I am going to be drowned—if I am going to be drowned, why in the name of the seven mad gods who rule the sea, was I allowed to come thus far and contemplate sand and trees?

Was I brought here merely to have my nose dragged away as I was about to nibble the sacred cheese of life?"

I learned in my grief months that life around me went on briskly, even as I limped through daily life and struggled to participate. "Funny they don't see us." It was not others' indifference to my battle that was disconcerting; it was that I could not engage in the life that surrounded me. Others were living their normal lives. They were walking on the beach and enjoying life. I felt excluded. Unlike the man in the open boat, fiercely trying to save himself, I was paralyzed to do anything to save myself from drowning. I was not rowing the boat or bailing the water. "Not living." I knew I had to reach the shore to save myself from drowning—to "nibble the sacred cheese of life". It was up to me to do something—to act! No one else could do it for me.

I figured out something else, too. Up until this time, my ability to act had been forced by problems or coached by others. I was not living my life, because the only life I knew was gone. I did not create my own life. I passively let other people create life for me.

For example, my friend planned a weekend trip for us to St. Pete during Adam's birthday month. I went—enticed to visit Chihuly art gallery. My sister encouraged me to plan a wedding shower for my nephew. I did—Breakfast at Tiffany's in an art museum. Adam's sister celebrated her 50th birthday in Charleston. I flew— because I knew Adam would have celebrated. All coached.

I reflected on my "not living" months. I had acted only once on my own in a way that invited a new experience. No other person coached me to act. I volunteered to sell meal tickets at a community spring fling picnic. It pales in comparison to my coached-life widow experiences, but it was monumentally important, proving that I could act all by myself to make change and let the new into my life. It took me six months to achieve that one progress. Six months!

As the school year neared its end, I decided I was ready to do something for myself. It was an intentional decision, as if I would choose between door number one or door number two; would you like a one week honeymoon or a six week honeymoon?

I had experienced the death of my husband, suffered grief, felt hollow, and lived isolated from the rest of the world for eight months. I had no idea exactly what I would do yet, but I had resolved to act. I would not go through the rest of my life in a state of existential nothingness. I was ready to put grief behind me by inviting change into my life.

It is this intentional declaration to act that will thrust you out of grief. It will happen when you decide you are ready to invite new things into your life, even if you are unsure what those changes will look like. It is your desire that will give you the power to act. It is a turning point.

I knew I had made some progress to live beyond grief. I had embraced and nurtured the memories of my life with Adam—stories I shared or held in my heart. Not only had I accepted Adam's death, I had also accepted that my life would never be the same. Life as I knew it did not exist, yet I sensed Adam's spirit was somehow part of my life, and that comforted me. With some coaching, I had gradually lived life. On my own I had invited at least one new thing into my life. I had "nibbled the sacred cheese of life". Now, I had intentionally declared to do something—to act—to live beyond grief.

I felt an awakening taking place. I felt empowered to release myself from the grief-fog—the "not living". I was beginning to "see clearly now". Grief slowly released its grip on my day to day life. I was beginning to feel normal again. I was winning the battle between "not living" and "deciding to act". I claimed this song:

I Can See Clearly Now

I can see clearly now the rain is gone.
I can see all obstacles in my way
Gone are the dark clouds that had me blind
It's gonna be a bright (bright) bright (bright)
Sun-Shiny day.
I think I can make it now, the pain is gone
All of the bad feelings have disappeared
Here is the rainbow I've been prayin' for
It's gonna be a bright (bright), bright (bright)
Sun-Shiny day.

from song by Johnny Nash

READER INVITATION: Think about the first months after your husband died. How did you react when friends offered condolences? Did an unexpected person care for your feeling of loss? Did you experience the inability to live a normal life? What was your daily routine? Did you encounter and solve difficult and unique problems? At any time did you feel like an angel lifted you? How did you feel when you observed others around you happily living their normal day to day lives? Are you gradually feeling ready to do something to win your battle against grief? Are you willing to invite changes into your life? To intentionally act?

NOW WRITE YOUR STORY:

No one else can define what your life changes beyond grief will be. I suggest observe what people do other than work. I also suggest continue doing what you did before you were widowed, if it makes you happy.

One thing I continued was to participate with my bookclub, a group of seven women I had known for twenty-five years. Books we read were as diverse as we were. We have read a book every six or seven weeks since 2002. Over eighteen years we have read roughly one hundred twenty-five books! And we have scrapbooks and FB posts of our reviews, our dinner evening photos, and our ratings for each book. That is a remarkable commitment on our part, and it is always an energetic fun-filled evening with friends.

Our very first book was <u>Last Train to Paradise.</u> One time we decided to theme our book <u>Devil in White City</u> with a trip to Chicago. I am still hopeful for a themed trip to Paris. After all, we did read <u>The Paris Wife;</u> <u>Mademoiselle Chanel: A Novel</u>; and <u>The Lost Girls of Paris.</u>

One book marked the days I became a widow, <u>WILD: From Lost to Found on the Pacific Trail</u> by Cheryl Strayed. Our book club hostess always themes dinner to the book, and gives an artifact related to the book. That night at book club the artifact next to my dinner plate was a framed quote from our book, <u>WILD</u>.

"Alone wasn't a room anymore,

but the whole wide world.

And now I was alone in that world,

occupying it in a way I never had before."

This was the quote I took home with me before the next morning's events would force me to admit my husband to Hospice care—my quote six days before I became a widow. It pretty much summed up where I was then. Alone.

I connect with books. Books take me places I will never go. Books create friendships. Books make me happy. So I stuck with my bookclub.

I added new activities to my life. These were small and simple changes, but things that were new to me—changes I made on my own to jump-start living again. I participated in group Sip'N Paint classes, sometimes with a friend and sometimes by myself. I liked it when the instructor said, "If you don't like how it looks, just drink more wine!" It made me laugh as I took another sip. I also took yoga class, but tired of it.

Much later, I took an interest in sports, especially basketball. I followed NBA games through the entire season. I once drove one hundred fifty miles to Miami to watch the Miami Heat play a Saturday afternoon post-season game against the Philadelphia 76ers, then drove back home. I had never been to an NBA game, and I wanted to see LeBron James play his last season in Miami. So I went. I ate fish tacos and drank a beer at the concession before game time while I people-watched. I took my end seat in the stands next to two men, a father and son, who ironically cheered the 76ers. I had a fun time. I was proud of myself for the courage to act and not to rely on another person to create my life for me.

One of my biggest changes came when I retired four years after my husband died. With extra time and new resources, I invested in a beach condo which gave me more days near my family, and a vacation share property on the side. The effort to furnish and decorate it afforded me a creative outlet, and I was happy during the entire process of setting and accomplishing a big goal—a goal I could never have come close to even imagining in the grief months— a goal I accomplished with the help of my new realtor friend, Cindy.

I have two widowed friends who made changes in their lives, too. Karen adopted a dog which became a loving part of her life. This was remarkable, since she was, and still is, a "cat lady". She also took private art lessons. She now teaches painting classes, and as an artist has recently showcased her work as a featured artist at a prominent mountain retreat in North Carolina where she bought a home and lives part time.

The other friend, Carol, joined a travel club. She made annual trips with this same group. Her experiences included trips to the Holy Land, Egypt,

Ireland and other interesting places. From these travels, she expanded her friendships and is now involved in social activities with them, like weekly card games and birthday parties. She also volunteered at her grandchildren's school. She continued her sailing life with all its regattas, commodore meetings, and pot-lucks. She even started an annual sailing race in memory of her husband.

My own mother, Rachel, after being widowed in her late seventies, once met at three different churches, because each of them offered a monthly program that gave her an uplifting social outlet. It delighted me that she went on a Caribbean cruise with one church group, a total departure from her previous life. She also hosted and participated in Game Fridays every week, playing Scrabble and Chicken Scratch dominoes with a group of women friends. These changes she made in her life made her happy.

Recently, a friend's ninety year old mother, a widow, moved to an independent living apartment, a change that simplifies her life, serves her meals in a dining room with linen tablecloths, and offers lifestyle activities. One of her first observations was that she would like to participate in the group exercise classes. She looked forward to making this change in her 90's life.

Making changes is part of reinventing your life. I shared several examples of how I made changes and how other widowed women I know made changes in their lives, too. For each one of us, we fought the battle between "not living" and "deciding to act". As a newly widowed woman, you have the same battle to fight. And, deep down, you know which one you want to win.

Your intentional desire to act and make changes, no matter your age, can help you choose your new life and end up happier. You do not have to remain stuck in "widow identity", the time between the death of your husband and your decision to act—to reinvent your life.

I'll never know, and neither will you, of the life you don't choose.
   from <u>The Beautiful Things</u> by Cheryl Strayed

CHAPTER 6

AWAKENING SEXUALITY

I had read Joan Didion's memoir about the death of her husband because I wanted to know how another woman experienced losing her husband. So I read with great interest. But I needed more.

Unexpectedly, reading a different widow's account, I did learn more. She described being with another man for the first time after many years. What was it like for this older widow to be with another man? It was awkward. It was not the same as being with her husband. Yet she reached out to satisfy her need for intimacy. I'm glad she included that part, because a widow needs to know.

There is no denying that the absence of physical touch and loss of emotional tenderness weigh heavy on a woman, no matter her age. I was not unlike this other woman. She had been married forty years. I had been married thirty years.

I followed through on my decision to act—to do something for myself—to put grief behind and claim living a normal life—to reinvent my life. I was not hesitant to go to a place I had been with Adam. In fact, I sought out places we had been because I felt connected to our past. Eight months had passed since he died. I decided to go to South Beach Miami. I had not been in several years; I was familiar with the area; and it was less than a three hour drive across Alligator Alley and south to Miami. I made reservation at the historic National Hotel—not a hotel where Adam and I had stayed, but next to the Delano with its white wafting floor to ceiling curtain walls—a place where we had celebrated more than once.

All I cared about was sitting by the iconic pool and sipping a pina colada. It had been a turbulent and tiring two years of illness and death and grief. Just the thought of getting away, experiencing a change of scenery, and being waited on made me happy.

As I drove under the hotel portico, my car radio began playing Rod Stewart's song "Forever Young". I sat stunned. I teared up. I had chosen this song to accompany Adam's memorial video. I felt hearing this song exactly when I arrived was more than a coincidence. It was a sign—a good omen that Adam somehow affirmed my new freedom. I listened to the entire song before handing over my key fob to the valet.

I felt joy for the first time in months. Real joy! Granted, a fabulous vacation experience awaited, but more than that, I was joyous because I had intentionally declared a change in my life. I had finally taken charge and acted. This was me beginning a life on the other side of grief.

What happened next was completely random and spontaneous. My second day there I got a text from my friend, James, asking how I was doing. We chatted, and because I knew he lived within an hour of Miami, I invited him to sit by the pool with me and have an early dinner the next day. I knew James' playful nature would make me laugh. I needed that. Although we talked occasionally, I hadn't seen James in a few years. I had known James for fourteen years. We met at a fitness gym and became friends. In fact, Adam knew James, too.

We had all gone to some music events together and he once spent a Thanksgiving morning at our house. I looked forward to James' company the next day—sitting by the pool, sipping summer cocktails, remembering old times, and catching up. I would not have to awkwardly eat dinner by myself.

James arrived at two o'clock. From my chaise at the far end of the pool, I saw him saunter down a palm-lined walkway and exude his confident self past a flirtatious couple in a cabana, and a chatty group in the pool. I had forgotten a man's look of health and walk of vigor.

Knowing James was there to spend time with me made me happy. I waved. He tipped his head back, smiled, and walked straight to me. My eyes were locked on him. I imagine others at the pool watched him, too. He was easy to look at, somewhat exotic, as he tossed his long, sleek, black hair away from his face. La bise and greetings. The "not so ordinary" had just nudged into my "not quite living yet" self.

Act I. We talked for two hours. Nothing was left unsaid. We laughed. The pool attendant served us

Cuba Libre and Pina Colada. At one point we ducked into a cabana to escape a summer rain shower. The pool afternoon gave way to a change of clothes and early dinner next door on the Delano Hotel pool terrace. Afterward, we sipped wine on my room's balcony overlooking the blue-lit pool. We talked. He lingered. It was life—not life on a shelf, but life as a two-act play with only two actors.

You know where this is going. I don't have to remind you that I had read a widow's account of being with another man for the first time after her husband's death—and it was awkward.

Act II. James spent the night with me. For the first time I felt alive again, no longer a fossilized sexual being. That's how I described my physical and emotional awakening. It was a beautiful, tender, caring night. Being held, touched, and caressed brought me back to life again. James was my healer. I was undead.

Pina Colada

2 oz. cream of coconut
2 oz. pineapple juice
1 ½ oz.light rum
2 cups ice
½ oz. dark rum
1 slice fresh pineapple
2 maraschino cherries
1 umbrella garnish

Place cream of coconut, pineapple juice, light rum, and ice in a blender. Pulse until smooth, then pour into a tall glass.

Top with dark rum floater and garnish with pineapple chunk and maraschino cherries skewered onto a paper umbrella.

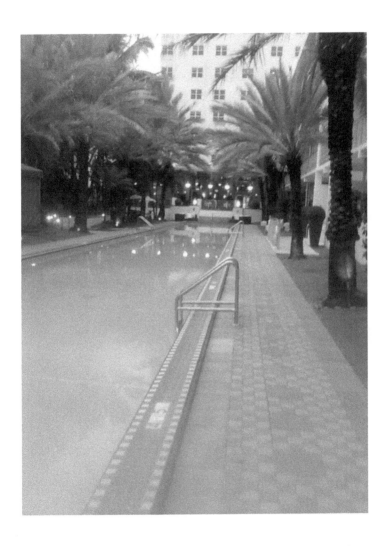

iconic pool at the National Hotel, Miami Beach

READER INVITATION: Think about your physical needs and sexuality. Are you expecting to one day meet someone you can be affectionate with? Or intimate with? Are you inhibited about your sexuality? Are you willing to take a risk by being with someone you already know? Are you curious about online dating? Do you know how to explore your sexuality in safe and healthy ways?

NOW WRITE YOUR EXPECTATIONS:

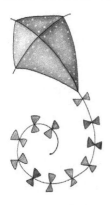

For me, intimacy further awakened the possibility that I could again begin to live a normal life. Two things precipitated this: One, I had already declared my intention to act—to put grief behind me and invite change into my life. Two, I now knew I was not afraid of intimacy.

You probably have a lot of unanswered questions. No two widow's experiences will be the same. What is the same is that you are a woman. A woman has specific needs for intimacy in a caring and loving relationship. But a woman can also explore meaningful relationships that will never be a marriage. Remember, the life you had no longer exists.

You can take charge of your intimate life. You can take charge of your affectionate life. You can take charge of your companionship life. Your level of desire will guide you.

The human heart is essentially romantic, and that is what makes the human being humane. Without romanticism, our life would be like a fossil.

Unknown

CHAPTER 7

SEEKING SPIRITUALITY

I had neglected my spiritual life. Although my background had been influenced by church and a religious family upbringing, I had not been true to that part of my life. My Christian beliefs had stagnated, and I found myself open to new ideas. I searched for deeper meaning in my life.

Reaching spiritual awareness is a very personal thing and is expressed in many ways. For example, in AA Twelve Steps, references to a "higher power" connote spirituality. In religions, the name and teachings of a God are revered. Whatever you call it—it's a conviction that outside of an individual exists a greater power of the universe. How one connects to that power is highly personal. For some it is through nature. For some it is through art. For some it is through religious teachings. For many it is elusive, never to be found.

My search took me to meditation, and I found the most welcoming young woman. She had just started her teachings on a You Tube channel.

I began Buddhist meditations with an Australian woman named Mindah. (Adam would have liked the Australian part; he had fond memories of living his teen years in Australia.) Her introduction and purposes were my first experiences of Episode One. It was perfect for me because I was a beginner. I knew very little about Buddhism, its teachings, or meditation.

Mindah was like a friend talking to me. Her sooth-ing accented voice calmed me. She was a great teacher, perfectly balancing her personal stories with teachings of Buddhism. She taught how to meditate, and the importance of the breath and breathing as a conscious awareness of the present moment—as an introspective spiritual practice. I would sit on my lanai and listen to Mindah's Buddhist teaching and follow her breathing meditations. It was all new to me. I felt a cleansed calm with each new episode.

I even joined a meditation group at the Unitarian church. I did not know anything about Unitarians except that Ralph Waldo Emerson, the American Transcendentalist essayist and poet, had been a Unitarian minister.

The Unitarian church meditation group met for an hour and a half one night a week. I knew no one. Anywhere from six to ten people attended. I had no idea what to expect, but I was willing to learn.

After a time of greeting and introductions, one "leader" read from a text—usually a poem or inspiring passage—followed by an invitation to meditate. A Buddhist chime would signal to begin and to end. We took turns being a leader.

Meditate meant close your eyes, empty your mind of all thoughts, think only of your breath in and out of your body, be fully in the present moment. At first I found it a bit uncomfortable to meditate in the presence of other people, but I soon learned to tune out my "monkey mind". I liked going. I looked forward to it, because honestly, sometimes it was the only group of people I had conversations with all week, and I always left feeling uplifted and happy.

I was still curious, so I read other Buddhist teachers. In my search for greater meaning, I became intent on following the details of an eight hour solo retreat, an entire day of meditation I had read about. Just me. At first, I didn't think I could do it. Eight hours is a long time! But when I read through all the ceremonial activities, I knew the time invested would inspire me. I valued ceremony, ritual, and symbolism.

My eight hour solo meditation retreat involved chanting, expressing gratitude, preparing a simple meal, taking a nature walk, writing in a journal, making a list of barriers. Two final rituals included burning that list in a flame and preserving the ashes, symbolic of releasing the past; then expressing gratitude for my life by counting out stone pebbles for each year lived, and also counting out pebbles for each anticipated year remaining. On each future birthday, gratitude would be expressed as one pebble was moved to the past. To me, these were powerful symbolic affirmations in my search for spirituality.

In preparation, I collected all the artifacts I would need. I bought a special nature journal with a seed pod pressed into the cover, and handmade paper pages bound by a twig. I identified the plate and bowl and cup I would use for a simple, mindful meal. I bought wildflower-like flowers and a bag of smooth pebbles. I set out a candle and a chime.

I did all this with great dedication. I felt this ritual would move me to a new place in my spiritual life and give me inner strength. It happened at just the right moment. I had grieved. I had acted in specific ways to make progress through the difficult eight months following Adam's death, and now I sought strength from outside of myself.

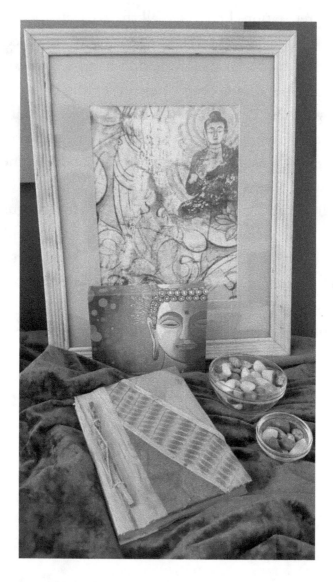

spiritual retreat journal and counted pebbles

These are the words I journaled in preparation for my eight hour spiritual retreat:

I am better than I was last week, and next week I will be better than I am now.

This is a journey. The journey is a river. The river is long. Follow the river.

This is part of a meditation affirmation I said during my spiritual retreat:

Aging Metta
The Prayer of Loving Kindness

As I grow older,
May I be kind to myself;
As I grow older,
May I accept joy and sorrow;
As I grow older,
May I be happy and at peace.

This is a higher-self affirmation I said at the end of my spiritual retreat:

Resting in Awareness

Rest in this state of being I have become. Let everything go. I am complete as I am. This is a complete surrender to that higher or deeper power that is always within me. I am it. It is me.

These are the final words I wrote in my spiritual retreat journal, recorded at 6:15 P.M.—nine hours after I started my solo meditation retreat.

Words of Buddha

"Don't believe it because you have read it or because I say it. Believe only because you have tried it and found out for yourself that it is true."

READER INVITATION: Think about your spirituality. Have you sought strength outside of yourself? Is spirituality something that's already part of your life? Do you already trust and believe in religious traditions from your past? Or is it something foreign to you? Do you wonder about spirituality or God or a higher power? Are you curious about meditation as a spiritual practice? Do you think rituals would add inner strength to your transitioning life?

NOW WRITE ABOUT YOUR SEARCH FOR
INNER STRENGTH:

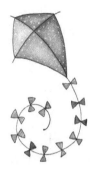

I had grieved two deaths—Adam's and mine. Life as I knew it was gone. I had remembered our stories of the past— meeting and marrying. I felt Adam's presence. I had spent eight months in grief and solitude before resolving to act—to do something to move forward. I had awakened my sexuality.

And now, in the same eighth month, I had applied deep spiritual practices to my stagnant soul. Beyond self-reliance, I could now rely on an enlightened inner strength. By this time, I was fully aware that I was in the process of actually reinventing my life. It felt so good to finally be on the other side of grief. I said "Goodbye" to my "widow identity".

My spiritual quest through Buddhism and meditation happened at the right moment. I learned from these teachings. I feel at peace knowing my widow's journey expanded to include a search beyond what was familiar. Teachings of Buddhism and meditations, as well as ceremonial rituals, met my need for deep spirituality at that one moment in time. My familiar religious roots could not speak to me in the same way.

Beyond those enlightening experiences, I later joined my heritage Christian church, reconnecting to my roots. Familiar liturgies, prayers, hymns, and scriptures augmented my spiritual quest. Church rituals gave me opportunities to honor Adam, too. At Christmas, those who lost a loved one placed a special memory ornament on a tree. And poinsettias and Easter lilies in memory of a loved one adorned my church in special seasons. These were simple but symbolic ways to honor the spirit of the dead among us.

Because I found the ceremonial and symbolic rituals of my spiritual retreat and church traditions to be important, I sought to create my own rituals of remembrance for Adam. I have found that the most meaningful way to honor the dead is to incorporate rituals that are personal. The date of birth and the date of death are the obvious markers of a life, but the dates of memories are the markers of a life lived, the most significant ones that deserve to be honored. Grief is often triggered by dates— anniversary dates, a birthday, and holidays. Rituals validate the grief that resides in you and resurfaces, especially on these marker dates.

I previously wrote about how special February thirteenth was, because it was the date Adam and I met. I always have a mix of sadness and happiness on that date. Sadness that Adam is gone; happiness that I recall joy.

My "progress journal" the first February 13th:

I have thought about our day we met almost all day. I knew it was going to be a day of loss for me, and it was. I tried to create some memories. I left work and bought a glass bead for my necklace—red and silver—to remember our February day—the day we met and flew kites. I also ate at our favorite waterfront restaurant, to sit outside and be near the water. I sat at the same table where we once sat. This was one of my rituals to remember the day we met.

On our wedding anniversary date, I go to a beach to watch the sunset. I relax in a chair with a glass of wine and listen to waves lapping the shore. Adam and I watched countless sunsets looking across the Gulf of Mexico to a vast horizon. Clouds made it even more perfect because light transitions painted the sky pink, lavender, yellow, and orange with each passing minute. If a clear horizon revealed, we watched for the green flash, an atmospheric phenomenon that flashes green at the second the last ray of sunlight disappears on the horizon. We saw it three times that I remember. *This is my ritual to honor my marriage with Adam.*

Making room for happiness does not mean that grief moves out. I keep a memory box of things that remind me of Adam's life. Some are photographs. Some are artifacts. Some he kept from his life before we married, and some I added from our shared life. On a day when I feel loss and grief, I will lovingly touch pieces of his life that remain as artifacts. He purposely saved them—like the list he wrote in blue ink before setting sail for his year of cruising the Abacos. He printed his list in familiar capital letters.

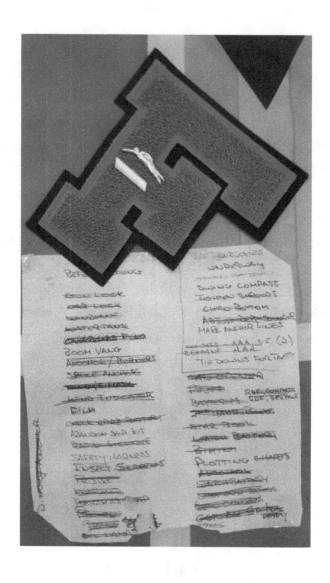

Adam's "BEFORE LEAVING" cruise list and high school letter with Swim Award

Many more things are written on Adam's cruise preparation list. I always feel connected to him when I read this, even though he cruised two years before we met. He talked about it many times as an adventurous part of his life. What I see when I touch and read this list is his attention to detail and his plan to reach a goal. I know he also made time for fun in his life—a Frisbee. I see his distinctive print writing. Other meaningful life events are inside this memory box I keep to see and touch Adam's life. I express gratitude for his life and for the days we shared our lives together. *This is my ritual to keep Adam's life close to my heart when I need tangible comfort.*

Finally, do not push back your feelings of loss on holidays. During the first year they are especially painful because the empty space is there for the first time, not only for you, but for family members. They grieve, too. Loss is silently broadcast out loud because it is so evident a loved one is missing on holidays.

Observe ways to unveil your thoughts about your absent husband instead of hiding them and awkwardly trying to be fully present in a family gathering. Light a candle in remembrance, say a prayer that honors his life, set his photograph on a table, propose a champagne toast, serve his favorite food—or even ask others to recall some special thing he said or did. These memories can be shared as part of a family tradition during part of the day. *These are some rituals to remember our holidays together.*

Rituals go back to ancient times, and are prominent in religious and spiritual ceremonies. These remembrance rituals enable me to honor my husband as part of my present. Like meditation, these rituals strengthen my inner being. Honor your husband with rituals that are personal and meaningful to you, especially on a day when a wave of grief laps the shore of your emotions.

There will be times when feelings of loss push aside your hard-fought happiness. And there are other times when grief and happiness live side by side. You learn to carry the weight of those feelings just like you are learning to act in ways that make room for happiness in your life. You will never feel happy all the time—but you will never feel sad all the time either. I have learned to live with grief. You will, too.

Grief never goes away; instead, it will share a space with other emotions in your life. You live with grief long enough that it slowly begins to thread its way into the fabric of your life. It is part of who you are now. You wear it bravely.

Early in my search to live beyond grief, I thought I could rid myself of grief. "I wanted to get rid of it!" I learned that does not happen; could not happen; should not happen. Grief is the "homeless dog" lingering under your porch. You may as well invite him in. (Levertov poem).

What I learned instead is that although grief resides in who I am, it does not define who I am. It was my intentional decision to act and invite change into my life that allowed me to gradually reinvent my life in ways that diminished my grief and made room for happiness; it was my spiritual quest that gave me inner strength to cope, and sparked meaningful ceremonial remembrance rituals. Wisdom I desperately needed early on, grew from my lived experiences.

Imprinted with your same loss, I offer you my own widow wisdom – nudging you to act in purposeful ways mindful of your happiness.

Ponder how these three things can make room for happiness to also dwell within your house of grief— spiritual questing, time, and wisdom:

- Spiritual questing grows your soul and gives inner strength.

- Time allows you to practice living without your husband. You get better at it.

- Wisdom carves essential truth from your own lived experiences.

The soulful poem, "Talking to Grief" by Denise Levertov, expresses so clearly how grief never really goes away. Learn to live with grief—as the "homeless dog" you bravely acknowledge and name. Instinctively, you know it will occupy a room in your house. Sometimes you go there. Sometimes grief opens the door and comes to you. Making room for happiness diminishes it.

Talking to Grief

Ah, Grief, I should not treat you
like a homeless dog
who comes to the back door
for a crust, for a meatless bone.
I should trust you.

I should coax you
into the house and give you
your own corner,
a worn mat to lie on,
your own water dish.

You think I don't know you've been living
under my porch.
You long for your real place to be readied
before winter comes.
You need your name, your collar and tag.
You need the right to warn off intruders,
to consider my house your own
and me your person
and yourself my own dog.

poem by Denise Levertov
used with copyright permission

CHAPTER 8

CLEANING HOUSE

It had been eighteen months since Adam died. By this time I felt clearheaded and unafraid to try new things. I was out and about fully engaged with life.

I spent extra time with friends and I explored on-line dating. I made new friendships that added a fresh dimension to my life. My life felt normal and I was happy except for one worry. I knew that my home would eventually become unmanageable for me by myself. This uncertainty troubled me and caused stress.

Five acres, a two-story barn, and a house—it was big, and even with my two dogs, it was lonely. Although I felt safe, I never liked arriving after dark. I knew I needed to sell it, and I wanted to move to a smaller house in a neighborhood closer to work. I also knew it would be difficult to sell. Who wants a five acre property? Little did I know the next reinvention of my life would arrive so unexpectedly.

One afternoon a truck entered my long drive and stopped at my side porch. I saw that it was a woman, so I stepped outside to ask if she needed help or if she was lost. I did not recognize her.

She asked if I was Adam's wife. This was eighteen months after Adam died! As it turned out, her young adult son, Brent, took care of my lawn and acreage maintenance. I never saw him because I was always at school during the day when he worked on the property.

Adam had given Brent one of his first jobs, when as a twelve year old kid he drove by on a golf cart and asked if he could mow our lawn. Adam said, "Write a proposal for me." Then he explained what a proposal was. That was Adam's lesson in running a business.

In our mailbox the next day, Adam found a piece of lined notebook paper with penciled written descriptions and prices. Years later, Adam gave support and business guidance when Brent started his very own lawn and tree maintenance company with professional equipment and several employees.

The woman expressed her gratitude that Adam had been such an important influence and good role model for her son, but eighteen months after Adam died, what she most wanted to tell me was a story about a kite—a kite.

When Adam was ill, he hired extra help on the property, including her daughter Tiff. I had met Tiff. She was a sweet girl, about twenty, and sensitive to Adam's illness. To cheer him up, she had given him her neon pink stuffed monkey with long Velcro arms that could wrap around his neck. I still have Adam's monkey.

The woman's story went something like this: One February day, without telling the two workers where they were going or why, they all got into the work truck. Adam carried a black bag. They followed his directions to a neighborhood field. They had no idea what was going on or why they were there. And they wondered, what was in the black bag? Then Adam unpacked the black bag and pulled out—a kite! This was a large trick kite, the two-handed kind you see on beaches that lift and dive and swoop wide. Adam gave some instructions for how to guide it, then they each took turns flying the kite as Adam looked on. They all celebrated with a childlike joy, laughing and flying a kite in a field.

This experience really meant something special to Tiff, who told this story to her mother like I am telling it to you. Tiff knew Adam was not feeling well, yet he had created an unexpected adventure shrouded in mystery that gave them all pleasure in the middle of their work day.

I did not know that story. It was a beautiful story. Tears welled up in my eyes, because I saw Adam and me flying kites the February day we met. It was the last happy life story Adam created, and the last unknown story about Adam I would ever be told—the kite in the field story.

As the woman was leaving, I inquired about Brent. She told me he was looking for rural property east of town. I seized that moment of opportunity to say, "Well Brent should consider buying my house, because I'm interested in selling it. After all, he knows my property better than anyone else."

That's literally all it took to begin the sale of my five acre property, two-story barn, and house.

I realized that selling my home would sever my past. This would be the most overwhelming thing I had done since Adam died. Like most people, a lifetime of things had accumulated. Going through all that stuff stirred up the memories I had put to rest. It was hard because I had to make decisions about what to keep, what to donate, and what to discard.

The barn was just like Adam had left it. So was his workshop. Radio Controlled airplanes and other hobbies; tools and equipment—neat and in their place. Part of me did not want to disturb it out of respect for Adam. But the other part of me wanted to plow through everything to claim my new life. Now I just needed to get through the difficult part one day at a time.

The hardest physical work I ever did was move. From April to June all I did when I got home from work was sort and pack things one box at a time until late at night. I was exhausted. Without the constant help of my best friend, Cathy, I could not have done it. I remember one early evening both of us just lying back on the deck of the lanai totally exhausted— hot, sweaty, and unable to lift one more thing.

My brother and nephew drove over a thousand miles from Ohio to do the heavy lifting and to transport most of Adam's tools and big equipment in a moving truck back to Ohio. They towed their car. This was a big sacrifice on their part to help me. My brother had checked on me regularly and helped in other ways, too. I love my brother and nephew for helping me.

In the middle of packing to move, I also had to make time to look for a new house. Actually, I found the search rejuvenating because I knew it meant a new life for me. I was ready. I bought the perfect smaller house with a fenced backyard in a neighborhood near my work. That was a happy, happy day. With lots of help, I did it! My new life had a new home.

All my furnishings were packed into three PODS and moved to my new house. I had given away as much as I could and discarded the rest. Before I left Erewhon, I walked the entire property and expressed gratitude for every space Adam and I had shared. It was our home. We had designed and built it, and had lived there "happily ever after 'til death do us part". We kept our promise to each other. I raised my arms to the sky in a powerful, yet surrendered gesture to say thank you for that significant part of my life, and for the hard-won happiness filling my new life.

Angel

There is an angel
Watching over you
in good times, trouble or stress.
His wings are wrapped 'round about
Whispering you are
Loved and blessed.

~Unknown

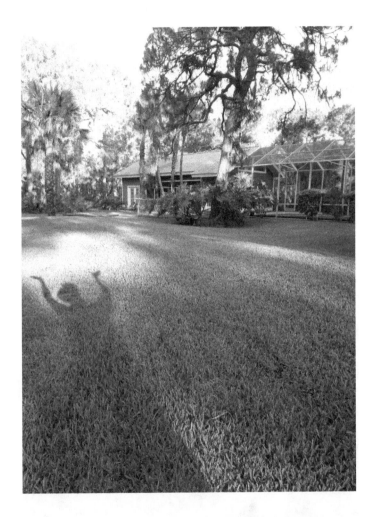

I raised my arms to the sky in a powerful yet surren-dered gesture, to say thank you for that significant part of my life at Erewhon, and for the hard-won happiness filling my new life.

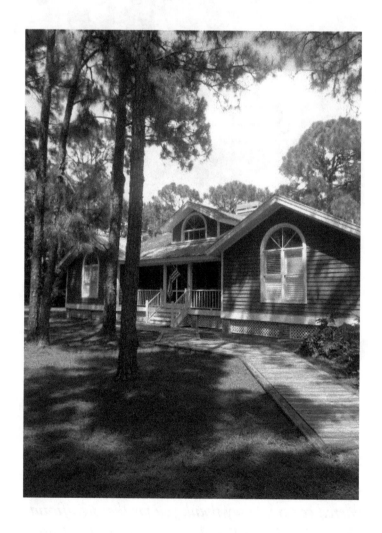

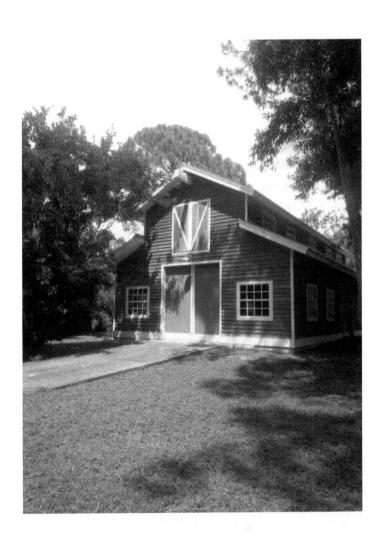

READER INVITATION: Think about where you live. Are you ready to "clean house"? Is selling your house an option? If you could move, where would you like to be? Near your work? Close to family in another city? In a small house or managed condo? Or an independent living apartment? If you cannot move, can you be diligent to "clean house" where you are? Can you simplify your life by donating and discarding things you do not use or need? Can you earnestly make room for your new life by "cleaning house"?

NOW T- CHART PROS AND CONS OF
MOVING TO A NEW HOME:

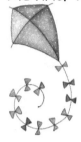

Widows get specific advice after their husband dies. One is not to make any big decisions at first. Moving would be at the top of that list! I think that is right, because you are already at a breaking point and need time to heal. Plus life is not normal yet. You do not know what you need.

But I would also shout, "Do it!" Don't postpone moving just because that is where you lived with your husband. That is not a good enough reason now. When you lived in the same house with your husband, you shared responsibilities. Your house was managed by both of you. Now you are the only one to manage your house. *Is your home too big?*

Most likely you, like me, will realize the large house will be too much for you. I had made repairs and improvements, and knew I would be managing an ongoing house maintenance schedule if I stayed there. I did not want that big responsibility as part of my life. *Are your house projects manageable?*

Are you already relying on your family to do everything for you? That would be assuming you have family that lives nearby who are willing, able, and cheerful to take on some responsibility for your big house maintenance. That is a lot for you to ask, however, because it alters their normal life with their own family. *Do you depend on family to manage your current home?*

Or maybe your family lives miles away from you, or your family lives in another state, or your family is not reliable, or you do not have family. These are all considerations that will shape your decision to move. *Would you move to a smaller, more manageable home? Or to a maintenance free condo?*

Move only if it makes YOU happy. Do not move if your only reason is to please other people. It would be a mistake if you left a perfectly well-suited and manageable home just to please someone else. But strongly consider "cleaning house" where you are. It will be personally cleansing, and it creates a space to welcome the new. *If you decide to continue living in your current home, will you take time to simplify by removing unused and unwanted items?*

At the same time, your children may be thinking long term. This is a valid consideration, so think about where you might future locate—when you will need hospitalization, rides to doctor appointments or to the hair stylist. *Would you relocate to another city?*

Eventually, you may need a two-part move—a move to a smaller, more manageable home now, while you are healthy and can independently manage a smaller home, and later, a move to an independent living apartment.

A small independent apartment removes all the worries of home ownership because everything is taken care of for you. You can even take advantage of meals served in a dining room, fitness classes, activity schedules, and concierge shopping services. Many new living centers have inviting courtyards, pools, gardens, and nature walks. A living arrangement like that is where I plan to move when I need help, and when I may need more levels of care. In fact, I have already toured one well known place in the area near where I currently live. I am not ready now, but at least I am giving it some thought for later. I will know when. *Later on, will you consider an independent living apartment?*

Even though none of us want to think about aging and being dependent, it is a good idea to think through these moving options at some point. When that time comes, you have already thought about it. You will have already visited sites and processed information. It will not be disconcerting to you. And it will be your idea—not an idea someone is forcing on you.

Downsize to simplify your life and get a new start. Moving to a more manageable home is a huge step in reinventing your life after the death of your husband. And it celebrates your independence and will to live in a strong way, so that you are not depending on others to create a life for you. You create your own life. And it frees your family to live their normal life, too.

Should I move or should I stay?

- Is your current home too big?

- Are your house projects manageable?

- Do you depend on family to manage your current home?

- Would you move to a smaller, more manageable home? Or to a maintenance free condo?

- If you decide to continue living in your current home, will you take time to simplify, by discarding unused, old, and unwanted items?

- Would you relocate to another city to be near family?

- Later on, would you consider an independent living apartment?

I remember when my mother moved to a smaller house. It was hard for her to leave her big two-story home where she lived many happy years with my father and raised four children. But I also know how happy my mother was in her new house, one that she could manage by herself and call home.

Moving to a new and smaller house helped me re-invent my life because it gave me a place to make into my very own. I discarded an accumulation of the old. I severed my physical past. My twenty month journey living beyond grief and reinventing my life resulted in hard-won happiness, for which I am deeply grateful.

I have never driven by my former home because I only want to remember it as it was when Adam and I lived there. To see changes or activity of others would alter my image of the past. I want my memory story of our home to remain pure.

You can't go home again.
from Look Homeward Angel
by Thomas Wolfe

I never named the woman who, out of the blue, appeared at my house eighteen months after Adam died to express gratitude and tell me a kite in the field story—the woman who made it possible for me to sell my house. She was an angel who appeared to me that afternoon. How else could I have been so blessed? I call her Angel. May there be angels in your life, too, as you act to move beyond grief and reinvent your life—inviting the new and making room for happiness

I no longer think of myself as a widow. My "widow identity" only occurred in the dark window of time after Adam's death and before I could act. It took time, but it also took brave determination to invite change as I reinvented my life to claim a normal life. I am living a happy life, and over time, with a widow's resolve you can, too! I wish you peace and joy on your widow journey beyond grief as you make room for happiness. I will end with a lullaby song I listened to before I fell asleep at night during those dark widow hours—when I needed a reminder to unfurrow my brow. It's "alright".

Alright for Now
Goodnight baby, sleep tight my love
May God watch over you from above…
So close your eyes
We're alright for now…
So sleep tight baby, unfurrow your brow
And know I love you,
we're alright for now

song by Tom Petty

FOCUSING...

Widow Wisdom:
How Grief Made Room For Happiness

- Embrace your memory stories. Tell them or hold them in your heart.

- Accept two deaths—your husband's and yours. Life as you knew it no longer exists, and it never will.

- Rethink group therapy when it augments your grief.

- Grief is "not living". Decide to act and make room for happiness.

- Awaken your sexuality. Do not be afraid of intimacy.

- Seek spirituality for inner strength.

- Clean house. Consider moving—to simplify your life and welcome the life you worked so hard to reinvent.

READER INVITATION: Think about these 7 purposeful actions mindful of your happiness. Have you already accomplished some of these actions? Are you slowly learning to live your newly widowed life? Is grief more behind you than in front of you? Have you taken actions other than these to begin to reinvent your life? Are you beginning to experience the gradual release of your "widow identity"? What action will you take next to make room for happiness and claim a normal life? Think of your newly widowed life as a house where, over time and with resolve, you gradually begin to make room for happiness. Although grief will always be a room in your house, you will no longer dwell there. Like the chambered nautilus "left the past year's dwelling for the new... and knew the old no more," you have the courage and resolve to create and go there too.

NOW, HOW ARE YOU BEGINNING TO MAKE
ROOM FOR HAPPINESS?

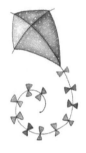

My Song Connections

Songs that give meaning to my own experience:

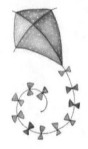

My Literature Connections
Stories, novels, poems, or quotes that give meaning
to my own experience:

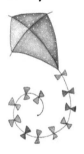

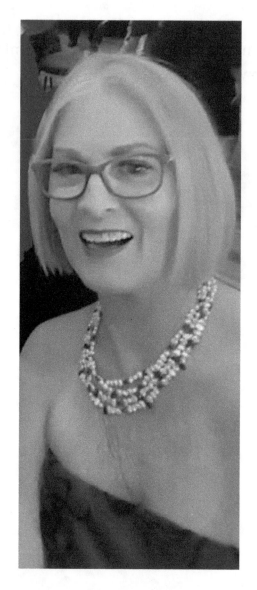

author, Ruth Rigby, the 7th year

ABOUT THE AUTHOR

Ruth Rigby lived the events of each chapter, then reflected on the process of reinventing her life. Remembering as if it were yesterday, the words of her story spilled out seven years later.

From the time she faced the death of her husband, Ruth knew she would one day write these events, not for herself, but for so many other women who were wife one minute and widow the next—women facing the same heartbreaking death of a husband, their grief, and their uncertain future— women who needed a wisdom to live their newly widowed life and be happier.

Ruth's interests are her two dogs, art, nature, basketball, and all things French. She lives near Florida beaches and North Carolina mountains.

A retired English teacher, Ruth graduated from University of North Carolina at Charlotte, B.A. and Georgia State University, M.Ed. and Florida Gulf Coast University, Ed. Leadership. She held governing positions in national, state, and local professional organizations and was published.

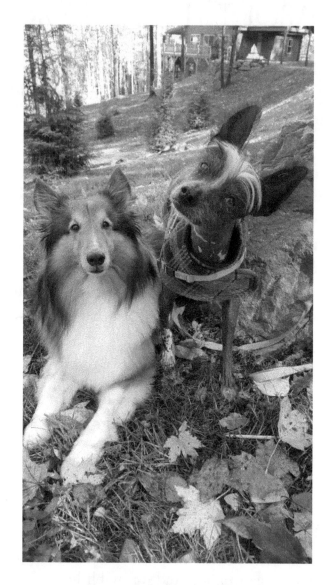

Google and Merlin, the 7th year

ACKNOWLEDGMENTS

Two close personal friends published their own books long before I did. My admiration for their perseverance and creativity decidedly influenced me to model their rigor and dedication to also write and publish.

- Thank you, Carol Fuery Ruot, for your enthusiastic encouragement, rounds of book talk, and faithful friendship.

- Thank you, Tony Neubroch, for being the poet in my life, and for sharing the language of your eternal soul in *A Feather's Touch*.

Two constant companions loved me unconditionally while I wrote in a spiral notebook, read memories from personal journals, reflected on a twenty month past, keyed all the words into a laptop, then revised and edited and sought publication.

- Thank you my Google Boy and Merlin Man, for reminding me it was time to Eat, Play, Walk!

RUTH E. RIGBY

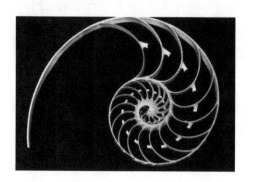

BIBLIOGRAPHY

Crane, Stephen. June 1898. "The Open Boat" N.Y.: Doubleday and McClure.

Didion, Joan. 2005. <u>A Year of Magical Thinking</u>. N.Y.: Harper Perennial.

Levertov, Denise. "Talking to Grief" in <u>POEMS 1972-1982</u>.copyright 1978 NY: New Directions Publishing Corp.

By Denise Levertov. From POEMS 1972-1982, copyright 1978 by Denise Levertov, Reprinted by permission of New Directions Publishing Corp., U.S. and its Territories rights only.

<u>The Poems of Emily Dickinson</u>, ed. by Thomas H. Johnson, Cambridge, Mass: The Belk-nap Press of Harvard University Press, Copyright 1951, 1955, 1979, 1983 by the President and Fellows of Harvard College.

Wharton, Edith. 1899. "A Journey" Ed. R.W.B. Lewis Vol. I. N.Y.: Charles Scribner's Sons.

FAIR USE LIMITED PORTIONS (IN ORDER)

Oliver Wendell Holmes, from "The Chambered Nautilus" (Public Domain)

Joan Didion. <u>The Year of Magical Thinking</u>.

Robert Stolorow, Ph.D . "emotionally dwell" in <u>Undergoing the Situation.</u>

C. S. Lewis. "invisible blanket" in <u>A Grief Observed</u>.

Nathaniel Hawthorne. "Act!" in <u>The Scarlet Letter.</u>

Emily Dickinson. 254 "Hope is the Thing with Feathers". (Public Domain)

William Faulkner. "The past is never dead." in <u>Requiem for a Nun.</u>

Edith Wharton. a wife's non-acceptance in "The Journey". (Public Domain)

Emily Dickinson. 1108 "The Bustle in a House". (Public Domain)

Bible. Psalm 23:4.

Beulah Malkin. "lovely things" in "Sanctum".

Steven Crane. "Funny they don't see us." in "The Open Boat". (Public Domain)

Johnny Nash. in song "I can See Clearly Now".

Cheryl Strayed. "alone in the world" in <u>WILD</u>.

Cheryl Strayed. "what you don't choose" in <u>The Beautiful Things.</u>

Unknown. "romantic/fossil" in Buddhist quote

Mindah-Lee Kumar. The Enthusiastic Buddhist. Youtube.

Unknown. In Buddhist quotes, prayers.

Denise Levertov. "homeless dog" (with permission, see Copyright page and Bibliography)

Unknown. "Angel"poem .

Thomas Wolfe. "You can't go home again." in <u>Look Homeward Angel</u>.

Tom Petty. in song "Alright for Now".

Crosby, Stills, Nash & Young. in song "Ohio".

THE KENT STATE SHOOTINGS:

Adam's Oral History

This is Adam's story—his eye witness account of the Kent State shootings on May 4, 1970. It was written by my high school student, Blythe Boden, from her oral history interview with my husband, Mr. Rigby (Adam). His oral history was part of "The War Years" research project in my Honors American Literature class.

The Weekend

Like many people Mr. Rigby was at Kent State for academics. He wasn't an active protester; he was just a curious onlooker. Prior to the killings there had been many uprisings at several college campuses around the country. The weekend before the shooting incident, many Kent State students had gone out to local bars, like college kids do, and gotten riled up. The mood was different this time, however. President Nixon had announced the invasion of Cambodia, and many students were upset at this decision. The Students for a Democratic Society (SDS) helped to start protests against the invasion. Fires were started downtown, and windows were broken. The day before the shootings, a Sunday, the National Guard was called out. Mr. Rigby remembers that Sunday as a quiet and peaceful day.

Monday, May 4, 1970
On Monday, May 4, Mr. Rigby heard rumors of a protest to be held at the commons on campus. This was a rally to protest the invasion of Cambodia. The National Guard stood high on a knoll. He thinks that it was so the guard could watch over the rally. He wanted to see the rally. He was an observer. Rumor spread of tear gas, so, like many other students, he brought a wet wash cloth with him—just in case. He remembers the people cheering as the rally started. The crowd was upset at the presence of the National Guard. Stones were thrown at the guard, so the students were dispersed with tear gas. He recalls it being smoky and that it was hard to see. He says chaos broke out. People were running around while the angry protesters charged the guards with rocks.

The Shooting

Supposedly a shot was fired, but he never heard this first shot. He saw the guard drop down and begin to fire. He was in their direct line. He remembers hearing and thinking that the bullets were blanks. He dove into a bush, hoping that it would be some sort of protection from the gunfire.

About twenty feet away from him, a male student was bleeding and screaming in pain. The young man had been hit in the buttocks. The bullet went in small, but came out through a hole the size of a grapefruit.

He remembers seeing several people on the ground. The protesting stopped. Mr. Rigby saw a girl sitting next to a guy who had been killed. She was shaking and crying. A guy who was carrying a peace flag dipped it into the bloody pool and began to wave it in the air. Mr. Rigby was splashed with blood from that flag.

Students Leave Campus

He returned to his dorm where he clicked on the radio and began taping the news flashes about the

Kent State shootings. Soon, the police arrived. All students were given one hour to get off campus. They weren't allowed back on campus for two months. He went home, which was two hundred miles away. All college courses were completed by correspondence.

FBI Searches Dorm

When he returned to Kent State months later, the dorm rooms were all torn apart. Students were told that it was done by the FBI. Any prescription drugs and questionable items were taken. Mr. Rigby's tape of the radio reports of the killings was gone, and he was unable to get it back.

The National Guard

The irony of the situation was that many members of the National Guard were college students, too. People signed up for the Guard in order to avoid being drafted to Vietnam. These people didn't want to go to war either.

Who was right? In this situation, I guess we'll never know. The protesters were wrong in throwing rocks, according to him. He also thinks that the invasion of Cambodia was wrong, so they had a right to protest. The Guard was wrong, too. They were untrained, and there should have been more control. He thinks that the Guard should have fired into the air, away from the students.

The Effects Afterward

This wasn't a happy time in the life of Mr. Rigby. He had a feeling of helplessness. He finished the spring quarter by taking correspondence courses, but he returned to Kent State for summer school. The campus was strange to him and he couldn't continue there, so he transferred to another college. He lost touch with the people at Kent State.

Mr. Rigby returned to Kent State only once—eight years after the killings. He went back to the commons where the protest had begun. He walked up to the hilltop where there is a large sculpture that is one-quarter of an inch thick. Bullets had gone through it. This time, there was a monument to the four students who were killed.

More to Adam's Story, by the author

My husband did return a second time to Kent State after that. We walked the campus knoll together and looked down toward the site of the killings, where permanent, lighted monuments are placed at the exact places where college students fell and died.

Ironically, the neighbor who lived across the street from my brother in Ohio when we made this return visit to Kent State, was one of those young National Guard that same day, May 4, 1970. One night during our Ohio visit, the Kent State student and the National Guardsman sat across the dinner table from each other and told their version of that fateful day decades ago, while our family listened to history.

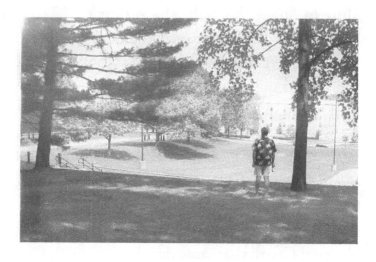

Adam looking from the Kent State University knoll where National Guard fired 67 shots over thirteen seconds. Memorial markers for the four slain students stand in the parking lot area where they fell. Nine others were wounded.

"Ohio"

Tin soldiers and Nixon coming,
We're finally on our own.
This summer I hear the drumming,
Four dead in Ohio.
Gotta get down to it
Soldiers are cutting us down
Should have been done long ago
What if you knew her
And found her dead on the ground
How can you run when you know?
　　　from song by Crosby, Stills, Nash, and Young

During that time of protest, the song "Ohio" was banned from being played on radio stations in Ohio.

Printed in the USA
CPSIA information can be obtained
at www.ICGtesting.com
LVHW011913270923
759473LV00006B/215

9 781638 371656